Additional copies of this book

REIKI FOR ANIMALS

and

REIKI PURE AND SIMPLE

available

Visit: www.secretgardenreiki.com

DEDICATION

To the "angels" in my life.
To my husband Jim,
four sons, and daughters-in-law.

To our grandchildren:
Abigaile, James, Ryan, Michael,
Amanda, John, Isabella,
Alex and Cameron.

They all fill my heart with such pride
and joy and I love them dearly.

Thanks to Amanda Sands, age 11, and Alex Sands, age 7,
for the cat and horse drawings on page 29,
and to Vicki Sands for her help in editing.

To Chris Rosenthal, my Reiki Master, mentor and friend.

And to the lineage Masters who have passed down their Reiki
instructions and knowledge...thank you!

To my family and friends for support and encouragement.

And to all the beautiful and special animal
friends who have been in our lives over the years
and given us such love and devotion.

Reiki will do so much
to help your animals in
so many ways.

INTRODUCTION

My name is Jeanne Marie Sands and I am a Reiki Master.

I have been doing Reiki and teaching it for several years and really enjoy this amazing and beautiful healing energy.

I love animals and decided that this book should be written to be used by my students and everyone who enjoys working with Reiki for animals.

My first book, Reiki Pure and Simple is the perfect introduction to the world of Reiki.
It will also introduce you to the wonderful Masters who are in my lineage (the direct line).

My lineage is: Usui, Hayashi, Takata, Gray, Rosenthal and I teach the Usui Shiki Ryoho method of Reiki.

I'm a proud member of The Reiki Alliance
www.reikialliance.org

Welcome to the world of
Universal Energy Healing for Animals

Reiki is healing energy
and can be given to anyone
or anything we touch.

BENEFITS OF REIKI FOR ANIMALS

Always remember to consult a veterinarian if your
animal has any health problems.

It is important for your animals to have regular
checkups with a veterinarian and to
make sure they have all the protection they
need against serious illness (such as rabies).
Reiki will help your animal in
many ways...here are just a few:

1. Hurt or sick.

2. Helps them to feel less pain.

3. Helps keep their bodies (and minds) balanced and strong.

4. More energy.

5. Heals feelings, fears, stress, and sadness.

6. Very relaxing.

7   Helps them to behave better, feel less nervous, calming.

8. Helps medicine and treatments to work better.

9. Before or after surgery.

10. Helps them to move better and be more flexible.

11. When they are in a show or competing, it will help them to listen, relax and perform better.

12. Reiki will help bring them to a place of comfort and love.

WHAT IS REIKI?

Reiki is healing energy and can
be given to anyone or anything we touch.

How does the word "Reiki" sound?

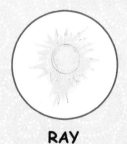

RAY

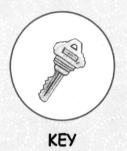

KEY

WHAT DOES REIKI MEAN?

Reiki is a Japanese word and means
knowing of the Vital Life Force which is the
energy in all living things.

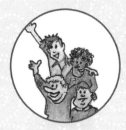

People

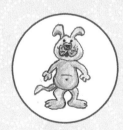

Animals

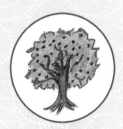

Trees/Plants

Reiki energy is everywhere
and always there
for us to use.

HOW DO WE GET REIKI?

Reiki Energy is
"everywhere" and
always there for us to use.

"UNIVERSAL ENERGY"

Try this:
Rub your hands together and then separate them.
Pretend you are holding an invisible ball.

As you move them away from each other
and back together...feel the

"ENERGY"

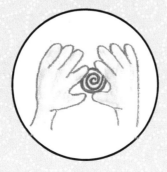

Your Reiki Master will open
the door for you to
Reiki Healing energy.

HOW DO WE PLUG INTO REIKI ENERGY?

We can tap into this universal energy to use for Reiki
healing after we have been "plugged in", or connected
by a Reiki Master using special symbols that
have been given from one master to another
and then to you.

The masters have been taught how to pass on this
energy so that it will be available to all of us.

This is done in a very special ritual, or ceremony,
through attunements, also known as initiations, and
are like special "keys" that open the door to
Reiki healing energy available to you always.

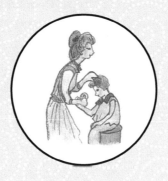

Always be super careful
when you are around
any animal.

IMPORTANT AND USEFUL INFORMATION

Always be super careful around any animal.

If they are not your pets, always ask for permission to touch them.

Not all animals like to be touched and that's o.k.

They will come near you when they are ready.

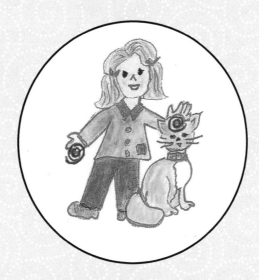

Animals have strong senses that they need to survive and may be really aware and careful of Reiki energy at first.

It may take time for them to get used to you and the energy but pretty soon they will come looking for you to touch them.

Do not try to come toward
or near an animal that you
do not know...especially if they
are not well or hurt.

HOW TO GIVE REIKI ENERGY TO ANIMALS

Remember that you must have permission before touching
any animal that is not your pet or that you do not know.

Do not try to come toward or near any animal that
you do not know...especially if it is not with their
owner or is alone.

Do not try to touch any animal who has been
injured, troubled. confused, or not well.

When you have permission, or if it is your pet, remember
that Reiki may be too much for them to
handle if they are not feeling good, or if they
are uncomfortable.

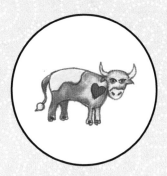

Many animals like shorter
Reiki treatments and
more often.

WHEN READY TO USE REIKI

Hold your hand out in a loving way (low and not
in their faces as they may think you could harm them).

Let them come to you and check you out.

Move slowly and do not force actions or movements on them...this could scare them.

They may "sniff" or "nudge" your hand...this is their way of getting to know you.

When they are ready, they will allow you to touch them and may rub
against you and either sniff or nudge your hands to invite you to
give them some beautiful and healing Reiki energy.

Sometimes, they just climb in your lap or lay down next to you.

If at any time the animal seems not to want Reiki,
please stop for now. Wait for a while until they are ready again.

Many animals like shorter treatments and more often.

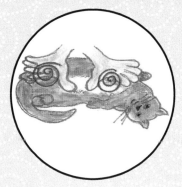

Reiki will help lessen pain
and speed up healing.
Remember to do the area
marked #3 on the chart
(stomach area) to help
with stress and to calm them.

REIKI WITH INJURIES

Giving Reiki right away after an injury will speed up the healing
and will help the animal feel less pain.

It is best not to touch the area of the injury or get too close to it...you
may leave your hands just above the area or you can "touch" them (if
they feel comfortable with you doing that) on other parts of their bodies.

The Reiki will get to the area that needs healing and will help comfort
them, help them get over being afraid, and feel your love.

Please try to remember to also give them Reiki on the area marked energy
point #3 on the chart (below the heart) to help them get over the
stress of getting the injury.

You may use one hand or both...it is up to you.
A small animal may like only one hand while a larger one may want both.

If an animal has been in pain or not feeling very well for a while, you will want
to give them Reiki often...the healing will take a little longer.

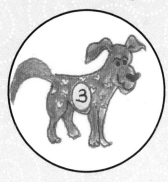

Always remember to give
them Reiki energy healing
on their ears.

DON'T FORGET THE ANIMALS "EARS"

Many animals love getting Reiki on their ears.
There are energy points located there too.

Actually, they also like Reiki anywhere behind
or under the ears as well.

Please be careful with the animal's tails...
they are sensitive and a very important
part of their bodies.

Please...always be gentle.

Always trust yourself and your
natural Reiki feelings...it is all good!

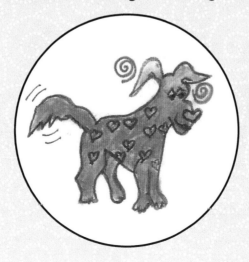

Reiki always goes where
it is needed and will
work on many levels...
body, feelings, thoughts, etc.

HOW DOES REIKI KNOW WHERE TO GO?

Reiki always goes where it is needed.

It is special and beautiful!

We do not have to think...it always knows
where it is needed and what to do.

It can heal on many levels.

Body

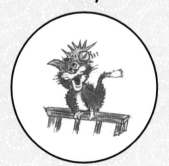

Mind (thinking)

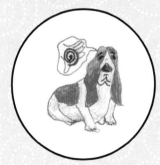

Feelings

Love

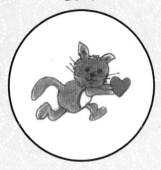

Fear

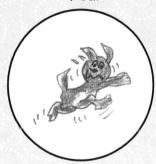

Sadness

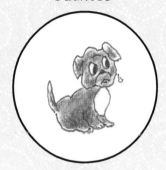

When an energy center is
not working well, an animal
may become ill or
be in pain.

HOW DO YOU KNOW WHICH ENERGY POINTS NEED REIKI?

(Always remember that Reiki given "anywhere" is always a good thing).

The best clues or signs to areas that may need Reiki help are:

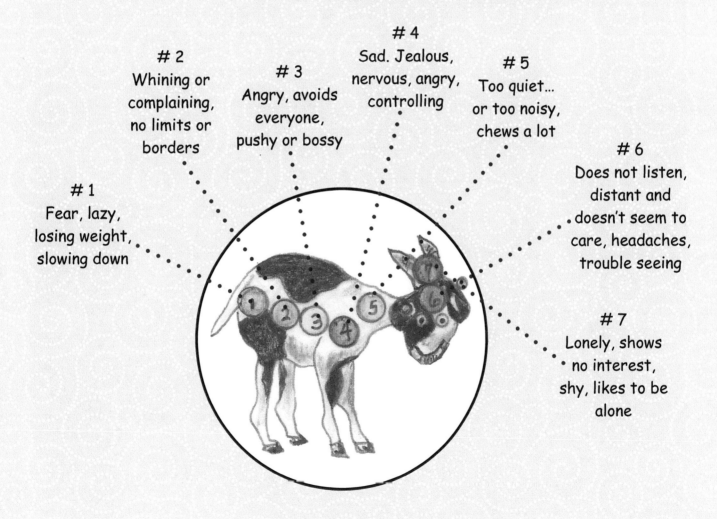

 # 1
Fear, lazy, losing weight, slowing down

 # 2
Whining or complaining, no limits or borders

 # 3
Angry, avoids everyone, pushy or bossy

 # 4
Sad. Jealous, nervous, angry, controlling

 # 5
Too quiet... or too noisy, chews a lot

 # 6
Does not listen, distant and doesn't seem to care, headaches, trouble seeing

 # 7
Lonely, shows no interest, shy, likes to be alone

There are seven Major energy
points and many more
Minor ones.

WHERE ARE THE ENERGY POINTS (CHAKRAS) FOUND?

There are many points, but these
are the important ones we will learn.

SEVEN MAJOR ENERGY POINTS
(IMPORTANT)

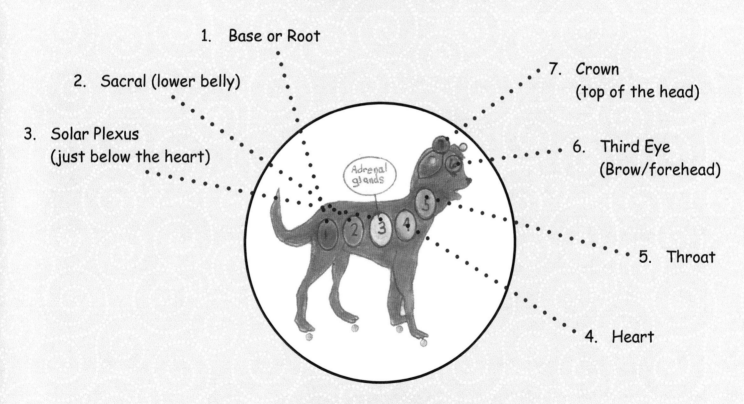

1. Base or Root

2. Sacral (lower belly)

3. Solar Plexus
   (just below the heart)

7. Crown
   (top of the head)

6. Third Eye
   (Brow/forehead)

5. Throat

4. Heart

Other energy points are:
4 paws
2 ears
And...there are 21 Minor (or less important) energy points.

Energy points are the same
in large or small animals.

28

ARE THE ENERGY POINTS THE SAME IN MOST ANIMALS?

Yes they are!
If you have other than four legged animals,
merely hold them (if you can) in your hands
and they will benefit from beautiful
Reiki healing energy.

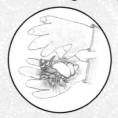

Reiki energy points are the same for any
size of animal...small or large.

Small

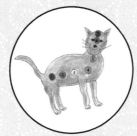

Large

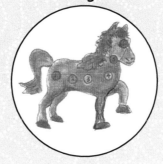

When animals are not well,
they sometimes will rub against
something to help them feel better.

SENSING WHERE REIKI ENERGY IS NEEDED

Animals have very strong senses.

They need these to survive.

Their energy centers are called chakras...pronounced Chuhk Ruh.

When animals are not well,
they sometimes will rub up against
something to help them feel better.

This is also comforting to them.

When a center or several centers are not working well,
they could become ill or in pain.

This is when it is important to give them Reiki, so the energy
will clear and heal these centers.

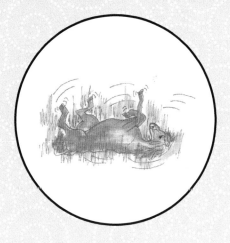

Reiki given anywhere on the
body is healing, beautiful
and a "good thing".